UNLEASH YOUR INNER PHOENIX

"THE ULTIMATE 7-STEP PERSONAL TRANSFORMATION FRAMEWORK FOR SMART WOMEN TO RADICALLY TRANSFORM THEIR HEALTH & LIFE."

KAVERI SEQUEIRA

First published by Busybird Publishing 2021

Copyright © 2021 Kaveri Sequeira

ISBN
978-1-922465-95-5 (paperback)
978-1-922465-96-2 (hardback)
978-1-922465-97-9 (ebook)

This work is copyright. Apart from any use permitted under the *Copyright Act 1968*, no part of this publication may be reproduced, stored in a retrieval system or transmitted in any form or by any means, electronic, mechanical, photocopying, recording or otherwise, without the prior written permission of Kaveri Sequeira.

Cover design: Busybird Publishing

Layout and typesetting: Busybird Publishing

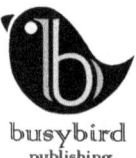

Busybird Publishing
2/118 Para Road
Montmorency, Victoria
Australia 3094
www.busybird.com.au

This book is dedicated to my son, Rafael, who means the world to me, and my two kittens, Emmy and Pixie.

Rafael is my purpose to be a better person, and my kittens never fail to inspire me every day.

About the Author

Kaveri is a certified WILDFIT coach who has been leading groups of people through the WILDFIT Challenge. She has successfully helped different clients achieve their transformation dreams.

This follows her health transformation with WILDFIT in 2019. When Kaveri discovered WILDFIT, it changed her life. She decided to become a certified coach to help other people achieve the same results. This coaching business is now her passion.

Kaveri is also an organisational change consultant and business strategist with more than fifteen years of experience in large organisations, including the top four banks/financial institutions in Australia – influencing operational efficiency, customer solutions and organisational growth.

In a person's transformation journey, Kaveri applies her knowledge for business transformation, as well as what she now knows about health and nutrition. She has studied Food as Medicine at Monash University, focusing on nutritional science. Kaveri is also a certified meditation and mindfulness coach, with a focus in yoga.

Get in touch

www.unleashyourinnerphoenix.com
www.foodfreedomwithkaveri.com
www.instagram.com/kaveri.sequeira/

Programs

Book a health game changer call
Try the WILDFIT 90-Day Challenge

WILDFIT Testimonials

Kaveri is an excellent, encouraging coach who was also a good example for us
– Lynette, Sydney, Australia

I feel the world should know more about WILDFIT and I am very grateful to have had Kaveri as my shining star leading the way. I will continue to use the new learned wisdom and apply this in my everyday life. Thanks WILDFIT and Kaveri for this amazing opportunity.
- Amanda from Berlin, Germany

It's been a great journey. Kaveri was an excellent coach.
- Anshu, Sydney, Australia

Kaveri has been a fantastic coach/mentor with my WILDFIT journey. Her commitment towards guiding us to a healthy lifestyle, constant support and guidance has helped me achieve the result I wanted, thus improving my overall health and fitness. Further, I am now equipped with the knowledge and tools to look after my own weight loss journey post WILDFIT. It's been a great journey with Kaveri and WILDFIT I highly recommend it.
– Avril, Sydney, Australia

My coach Kaveri answered all queries with patience and enthusiasm
– Parnell, Goa, India

I loved the program, and my coach Kaveri was so good at always keeping us motivated. WILDFIT has changed my life and I cannot be more thankful to Eric, Kaveri and everyone involved for taking me on this journey. I have entirely changed the way I eat, and I intend to continue to live WILDFIT.
– Taranna, India

Contents

Introduction   1

Chapter 1   3
The Message is in the 'Mess'
    The P.H.O.E.N.I.X. Framework   7

Chapter 2   9
The P.H.O.E.N.I.X Journey

Chapter 3   11
P for Powerful Awakening

Chapter 4   19
H for Hyper Inner-Vibe Audit

Chapter 5   31
O for Open New Pathways

Chapter 6   37
E for Energy Rising

Chapter 7   43
N for Not Giving Up

Chapter 8   49
I for 'I am at the Next Level'

Chapter 9   59
X for Xtra Acceleration

Chapter 10   65
Phoenix Rising – My Call to Be a WILDFIT Coach

Chapter 11   71
Boost The Lives of Others, One Person at a Time

Chapter 12   77
Spark Action for Your Success

Acknowledgements   85
Notes   89

Introduction

This book aims to help people using the successful P.H.O.E.N.I.X. Framework, which can be applied to any problem or situation in life. This framework aims to inspire people to have a radical shift in their life and their health to get it back on track – to help you achieve personal transformation and have a rebirth, just like a mythical phoenix.

I will be sharing the story of my transformation and how I turned my life around. It all started with getting my health in order. Health always comes first, and improving this area is vital as it impacts every aspect of your life. If this part of your life is great, you can have a million dreams – and if you don't have it, you can only have one dream! Health is wealth. My mission is to help one million people to improve their energy, vitality and feel amazing!

This book has activities and templates that will help you work through the steps in the P.H.O.E.N.I.X. Framework to achieve your goals and discover your purpose as to why you are reading this book. It will help you assess your priorities and look at what you are happy or unhappy about in your life.

This book can be used as a living journal and can be helpful whilst you are working through your goals. It can be a resource you use even after you have finished the book. I wanted this to be a something you can always refer to on your lifelong journey.

Who is this book for?

This book is for people who are willing to take responsibility for their lives, no matter where they are right now. If you know that you need to make changes in certain areas and you're struggling to do so, this is the book for you. It's for people who want to design their own goals and outcomes, then change the trajectory of their life in a positive direction.

If you know what it's like to have a yo-yo diet and not have any permanent changes then this book is for you. If you want to revamp their health and other areas of their life, like family, relationships, connection, career, business, finances and so on.

After reading this book, I hope you'll be inspired to act, to implement the P.H.O.E.N.I.X. Framework in your life and have fantastic success.

I would love to hear how you go. Please drop me a note through my website, Facebook or Instagram. Remember, it's all a journey, and you will succeed with this framework. It works. I am here for you and can't wait to see you unleash your Inner Phoenix.

Chapter 1

The Message is in the 'Mess'

"These pains you feel are messengers. Listen to them." - Rumi

When I say the message is in the 'mess', what I mean is that the events or circumstances we perceive as bad in our life (in other words, the 'mess') might be happening to deliver an important message for us to listen to and learn from. I am not saying these events don't make us sad or angry, but it might be an opportunity to look beyond what's going on and see the real message that life has in store for us.

Everything that has happened in your life decides who you are. Every experience I've been through has brought me to this stage, and I would not be the same person if I hadn't had those experiences. Those experiences taught me to do things differently and interact with people in a certain way. Nothing is a waste. There are no spare wheels in the universe. This is about acknowledging where you come from, and being understanding, kind and loving to yourself about what has happened so far.

Experience also gives you an idea of why you're doing what you're doing and why these things might have happened. You have to provide the experience with an empowering meaning and then take responsibility for it.

I didn't always have the point of view that I just described. I always thought, Why me? Why is this happening to me? But I feel all those experiences have sort of been a call to adventure. Joseph Campbell says that, as part of the Hero's Journey, the main character or protagonist is called to go on an adventure, facing many challenges, and comes home changed or transformed. If you're familiar with the journey, you'll know the protagonist has no idea of what is about to happen to them. They are mostly faced with challenges they need to rise to. Think Harry Potter, think Frodo from Lord of the Rings – you get the drift.

In these challenges, the protagonist needs to deal with the impossible. They try to deny it at first. Still, they accept the call to adventure, find a mentor to help them overcome their difficulties, then transform as a result of going through this experience. In the end, they achieve success in the mission.

My point is that you are the protagonist in your life. None of your experiences are a waste, and everything that has happened to you is a part of who you are. In some life stages, you may not be in the right place just yet, and you need to learn about moving forward from that place. You have to do the inner work so that you won't get stuck. You could be stuck in that pain, the vicious cycle of no progress, frustration, anxiety, sadness and loneliness – all of which I've been through, too, which is why I am delighted you have chosen to read this book. I believe the framework outlined here will help you move from your current state to the future, wherever that may be for you.

I grew up in India, and life was not very rosy. I wasn't born into a wealthy family, and money was always an issue whilst growing up. I was working very hard in a job that wasn't going to lead to any amazing future that I'd dreamed about.

I had visited Australia in 1995 with my family and loved it, so I knew immediately that I wanted to live in this beautiful country. My ex-husband and I started making plans to move to Australia, and we moved here in the early 2000s with barely anything to our names. We came with $2,000 Australian dollars and started from scratch. I was working a low paying job, my ex-husband was studying, and we really didn't have much at all.

I remember the first night we moved into our rented place. It was a cold Melbourne winter, and we had dinner with basically a slice of bread and French onion dip. I remember looking up at the ceiling, and there were glow-in-the-dark stars. We couldn't get the heater started because we did not know how. We also had this one blanket I got from my mum's friend.

I told myself I would remember this night and we would make it in Australia. After all, we'd decided to come here to make a better life for ourselves, and we had no idea what the journey would be like. It was hard to be without family and friends in a completely new place, but we were warmly accepted in Australia.

Fast forward a couple of years after our relocation to Australia. I had a great job and my career was progressing fast. Everything was going okay – we were coping, chipping away at our goals.

Then I got the worst news. I remember it was a Monday night, and I had a very uneasy feeling around 6pm. I just remembered not feeling right that evening. I had a meal with a friend at about 8pm, then came to the train station to meet my husband, who was suddenly being too nice to me. I felt it was bizarre because he wanted us to get a drink, which we would never do on a Monday night.

Anyway, when we got home, he sat me down near the heater and told me that my brother had been in a road accident and he didn't make it. I was totally shocked and confused. I asked if he was saying my brother was dead, and he said, *"Yes."* From that instant, my life changed forever. I had to speak to my parents, and they were devastated. No one was expecting that to happen, and it was a big transformational moment in my life.

I decided that life is too fragile and short, and I needed to make the most of it. I chose to live my life to the fullest and make every moment count. That is why I probably have so much drive.

I miss my brother. I've had a lot of grief and I know he will always be in my heart, even though it's been fifteen years. I know that day changed me forever. I was never the same person again, and of course it had implications on my relationships, too. I was so sad and lonely because he was my only sibling.

You should always keep in mind that 'your mess is your message.' After I lost my brother, I made certain decisions around how I want to live my life. If I had not experienced loss like this, I might have continued taking life for granted.

The other big thing that brought me onto this whole path was when my husband and I were trying to conceive, and I was told I was overweight. After my brother died, I put on a lot of weight due to emotional eating. I had no concept of what nutrition was. I also had all these hormonal imbalances, so it wasn't uncommon for me to put on weight.

I was trying to conceive but, obviously, that wasn't working. I went to three different specialists, and they said I had to lose weight, but nobody told me how. However, the third specialist told me I was infertile, and the only option was to do IVF. That really threw me off. As a woman, you're always told you're here to create and reproduce, and in my mind it was a basic thing every woman should be able to do.

At the age of 28, I couldn't conceive naturally, and that of course put a lot of pressure on my marriage. At the time, I decided no one was going to tell me something was impossible. I decided to accept the diagnosis, but not the prognosis. I knew I could change this outcome. I wasn't going to give up and take no for an answer.

I am thrilled to share with you that I did lose weight and went to a couple of other specialists. After some months, I fell pregnant naturally with my beautiful son, Rafael, who is now eight years old as I write this book.

Unfortunately, my marriage broke down in the end. I learnt a lot of lessons after losing my marriage. That long-term relationship ended in 2018, and I realised I was single, alone, and no longer sure of who I was. During the marriage, I just went along with things to achieve our family goals. We did okay work-wise and financially, but the relationship really affected me emotionally. My life was absolutely in shambles, but here I am. This was my mess, and there was a message in it.

This is my opportunity to share the framework I retrospectively applied to come out of that mess. In summary, don't ignore your past or belittle your life experiences. They are what make you who you are. It's also important to know that it's okay if you feel you can't see your deeper message. The framework will show you what that is.

If you would like to move forward, the one thing you need to do is accept where you are at that moment. Surrender to it as it's already happened. You cannot change it. There's no sense in resisting. The acceptance won't be forever. Resistance changes nothing and does not help.

Some people say they have too many limitations and disabilities to make the change, and that nothing they try works. However, as one of my mentors always says, *"It's not about the resource, but about how resourceful you are."*

Embrace the journey and let me show you the framework I used to work through and navigate some of the biggest transitions in my life. Trust me when I say the other side is amazing. It's well worth the effort.

The P.H.O.E.N.I.X. Framework

The Ultimate Seven Step Framework for Smart Women Who Want to Improve Their Health and Transform Their Life Radically

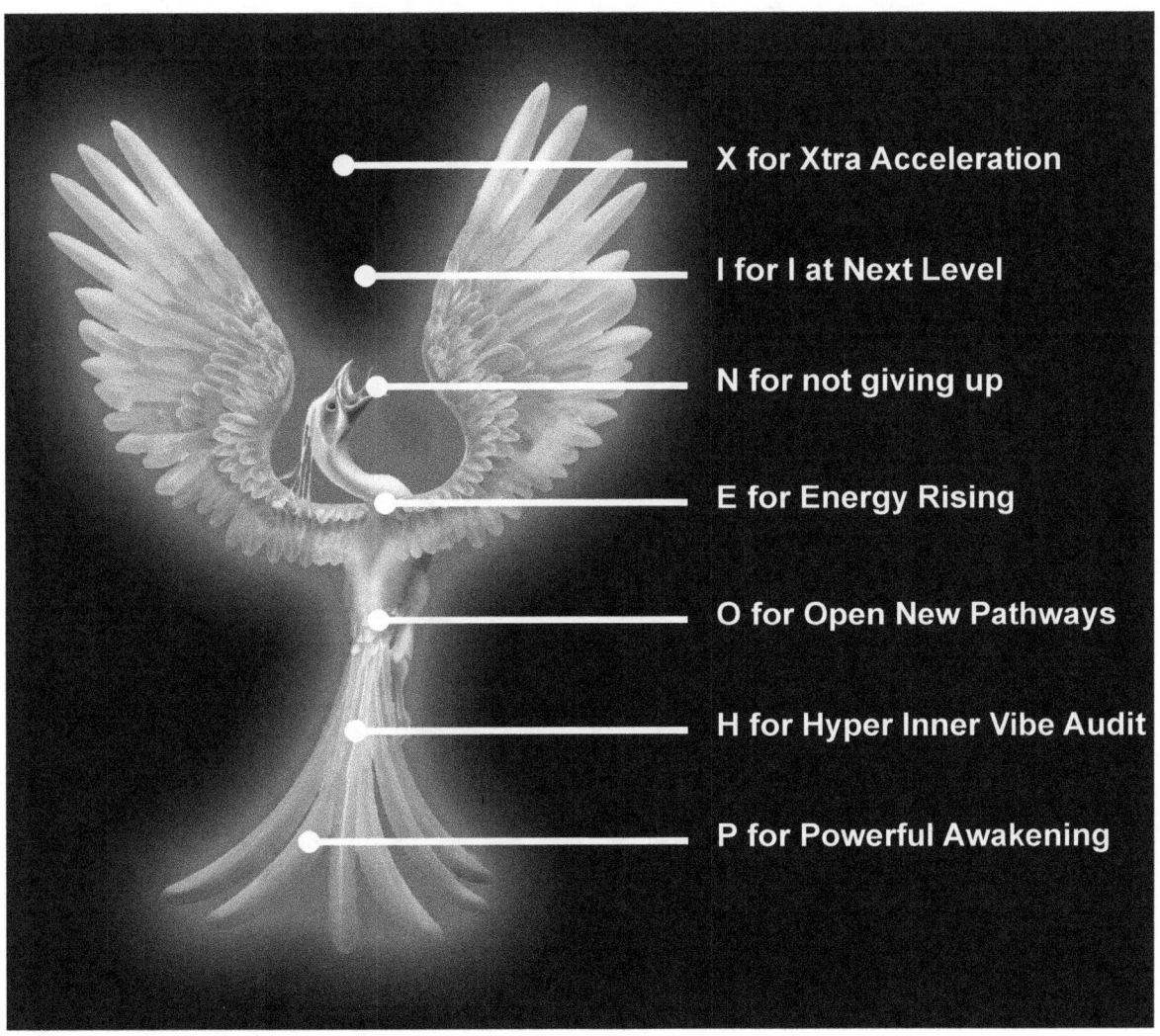

- X for Xtra Acceleration
- I for I at Next Level
- N for not giving up
- E for Energy Rising
- O for Open New Pathways
- H for Hyper Inner Vibe Audit
- P for Powerful Awakening

There are seven steps in the framework. However, it all starts with the very first step, and that is 'P' for Powerful Awakening (see Chapter 2).

I didn't see it coming, and I didn't know where it was going to take me. But I decided and chose to embrace the journey unfolding in front of me, and I am inviting you to do the same.

Of course, I know you will take the next step, as you have chosen to read this book, so congratulations. Go on – I'm cheering you on!

Chapter 2

The P.H.O.E.N.I.X Journey

"What you seek is seeking you."- Rumi.

I was waiting at the traffic lights one afternoon to pick my son up from school, and the realisation suddenly hit me. Every change I'd ever navigated through, every problem I'd solved, had basically come down to what is now the seven steps of the P.H.O.E.N.I.X. Framework. When I looked back, the steps were consistent – no matter the nature of the problem.

I decided that this is a framework I wanted to share with the world, especially if you want to transform your life, your health, and any other aspect of your life you are unhappy with. This framework can be applied to any problem, and you should listen to the insights that come from within.

So why is this framework important?

It gives you a step-by-step process that you can follow every time you are going through a transformation. It gives you practical tips, templates and activities that you can use to help change the course of your life's journey for good. It is useful for your health, and any issue or problem you need to find a pathway through.

I can tell you that the process works, and it's definitely a framework with a supportive structure. Remember, if you change nothing, if you don't do the steps, nothing will change. From my experience, I can guarantee that it will work if the steps are duly followed.

Therefore, this P.H.O.E.N.I.X. Framework is the ultimate seven step framework for personal transformation. However, I believe health is the most crucial aspect that you should start working on, regardless of your goal. We'll dwell more on that later.

I like the term 'P.H.O.E.N.I.X. Transformation' due to what the phoenix symbolises. I've always been attracted to the phoenix. Essentially this is an amazing mythical creature that turns to ashes when it dies, then transforms itself, reborn again in large flames. It's a real transformation, and you need to experience that kind of change where you basically dissolve your past self and recreate your future self the way you want. That is what evolution is.

Why have a framework around the phoenix symbolism?

There are many stages in our journey in life where we face struggles, then we evolve if we choose to. Our decision gets us to the next level of our evolution. We are called to step up and grow outside our comfort zone in order to achieve our goals. I feel you can have a much more fulfilling life if you embrace the challenges and struggles, even anticipate them.

You can use this proven P.H.O.E.N.I.X. Framework to help you become the new version of yourself. This book's content is an example of how I approached my recent health transformation, and it works. But if you don't implement the framework, you won't have the desired results. You need to understand and accept that this is an active journey that requires commitment. You just have to get curious about the framework, and I strongly encourage you to do that. Remember, this is a journey of self-discovery, and you can't change something you are not aware of. Get curious about truly knowing yourself.

Professionally, I am an organisational change manager, and I work with people and processes. The P.H.O.E.N.I.X. Framework is my model. I have used and applied it in integrating my professional expertise. It has certainly helped me in my transformation.

Chapter 3

P for Powerful Awakening

*"Yesterday, I was clever, so I wanted to change the world.
Today, I am wise, so I change myself."- Rumi.*

A "powerful awakening" typically refers to the biggest setbacks you have in your life. The biggest traumas you go through are the universe's way of getting your attention. You're pushed into a place where you need to reflect and make a new plan. In that reflection, you find insights that will help guide your path.

That is the first step in the P.H.O.E.N.I.X. Framework. You basically learn how you can tune into those insights, and you discover more of who you are.

How do you know if occurrences are supposed to be good or bad?

On reflection, sometimes the worst experiences turn out to be some of the best things to ever happen to you. That's what I found when I entered one of my biggest awakenings. For me, these were matters to do with my health and my relationship breakdown. I indeed found my purpose from some of the biggest traumas and worst experiences I've had in my life. The biggest mystery of human existence lies in not just staying alive, but finding something to live for.

This is what we will be talking about a lot more in this book. We have to look towards the pain, not away from it, because it opens a powerful portal. You get the answers from within, but we often don't pay attention to those traumas and pains. In fact, we do our best to avoid them. We seek pleasure and avoid pain, but I suggest we turn towards our pain and try and understand what it's trying to tell us. Ask yourself:

- **What is really happening?**
- **What is hurting me?**
- **What is true?**
- **Who are you?**
- **What is important to you in terms of your wants and needs?**

Then you'll learn a lot more. If there's a small voice that's been annoying you, pay attention to that voice. Pay attention and listen, because it carries the truth in it.

Losing my brother in 2005 had one of the biggest life-changing effects on my life. It was so painful. I experienced so much grief, but at that moment, when I was tuning in, I made some big decisions. After losing my brother, I was smoking twenty cigarettes a day. I was overweight and there I was, trying to fall pregnant. I was thinking about having a child and smoking away to glory. My brother had quit smoking a couple of months before he died. I had so many thoughts about him, but I thought, *okay, if my 22-year-old brother could stop smoking cold turkey, why can't I?*

My health improved because I stopped smoking. I didn't really need a cigarette, and it was ruining my health. That could have been an awakening I might have never had if my brother was alive, and I might still be smoking today. That's just one of the good things that came out of it. I'm not saying it was good that he died, but my point is that it was one of the good things that came out of me going inward and turning towards the grief I felt. Looking at my brother's life, celebrating and remembering what he has achieved in his short life, helped me realise that I needed to quit smoking.

Then there was WILDFIT.

I was first introduced to WILDFIT when I stumbled upon a masterclass by Eric Edmeades on the internet. What he said there just made so much sense, and so I just signed up for the WILDFIT 90-day Challenge. I moved from being unhealthy, overweight and having all these yo-yo diets and hormonal imbalances to losing fifteen kilos, having amazing energy and dropping my medication, among other things. It completely changed my life, so much that I decided to become a coach for WILDFIT to help others with their health struggles.

When WILDFIT entered my life, it was a very dark moment. I still remember the day I was sitting in my room. It was cold; it was winter in June. My relationship with my husband had broken down, and he moved out of the house two years before that. I actually liked someone else at the time and was hoping it would work out with him; I believed he was my twin flame. However, he had indicated that wouldn't be the case, and at that point, I was sitting in my room, completely broken and shattered.

I had thoughts running through my mind like, *"I am an amazing person. I know I am loving, caring and a good woman. I trusted someone with my feelings, and I was rejected. I felt I wasn't taken seriously, and I don't ever want to feel that way again."* As I was sitting in my victim mode, I was lonely, sad and grieving multiple losses.

At one point, I just looked up and said, *"I can't go on suffering like this. The pain has already happened, and now I am choosing to suffer because of it. How long am I going to sit in suffering? Why are you moping? Why are you beating yourself about it? What else could you be doing?"*

At that moment, I made a life-changing decision – that I would never allow myself to be treated poorly by a man again, and I would never treat myself so poorly that I would land myself in such a situation.

I decided to focus on what I needed to change my life and my life's direction. I was physically sick and unhealthy, and that made me take different medications. I was overweight and going to personal training, yet nothing was working.

I said to myself, *"You know, this is it."* This is the awakening I'd had – that my relationships, external world and the health results I was manifesting were not what I wanted. I wasn't where I wanted to be.

To turn this around, the first thing I needed to do was focus on my health. Everything was falling apart, and I didn't have the energy I wanted. I wasn't getting the goals I was visualising in my head. I wasn't manifesting it in real life. I needed to go within, and look at why this was happening. Fixing my health would give me the energy and inspiration I needed to turn every other aspect of my life around.

I started doing some research and stumbled upon a masterclass with Eric Edmeades, the founder of WILDFIT. What he said in that masterclass was so valuable. I decided to sign up for the WILDFIT 90-Day Challenge, and I am glad I did! I'd been in so much pain. I was just sick and tired of being rejected. I wasn't excited about too much in my life. I was just on autopilot. When I decided to focus on my health and had this awakening, I felt a sense of purpose. For the first time in a long while, I was putting myself first and prioritising my health.

I was also taking responsibility for my relationships. Obviously, there was some truth to why I wasn't the right person for that individual. It wasn't even about them, though – it was about *me* and being the best version of myself that I could be. I started asking myself, *"Are you giving yourself the best chance to be successful at what you want to achieve in your life, your health, finances, career and business?"* The answer was, "No, I'm not." That right there was the awakening.

One of the biggest things I felt insecure about was my health and the way I looked. I was stuck in a place where I did not know what to do. I was not getting the results I wanted. Once I joined WILDFIT, in ninety days I completely changed the direction of my health. During the challenge I lost eight kilos, which I had not done in years. All the pregnancy weight I'd put on dropped off, and I was in a place where I knew it would be a permanent change. After that, I continued to lose about fifteen kilos in total.

Now that I had my nutrition in control, it made sense to start personal training, and I found myself a fantastic role model who helped me continue to transform my body and life. This powerful awakening was very painful, but it gave me a better result with my health.

I can give you another example of a powerful awakening from when I was earning a lot of money. When I was in the marriage, we had accumulated debts for a mortgage, cars and things I bought for retail therapy. I tried to meet my needs emotionally by doing a lot of shopping. There was a lot of debt on my credit card.

After I did the WILDFIT 90-day Challenge, I realised I wanted to be a WILDFIT coach. I found it very difficult to make the decision due to the financial considerations, and it was going to be a significant investment. Still, I had a guided moment where I thought,

"Okay. If I can have this result with my health, there must be something to it. I need to do something about this intention of becoming a WILDFIT coach."

The opportunity came up, and I struggled financially to find the money to invest in the course. It was quite expensive, considering all the other debt I had. I was not getting any support financially as I had to make it work on a single mother's income. But I knew that I needed to do this WILDFIT coaching course, so I negotiated better payment terms on the coaching program fees, then reached out and asked a family member for help. At first, they said yes and I committed to the course, but when the time came, they said they could not help after all.

This was another powerful awakening. I felt so hurt and traumatised that I was in this position. I felt so let down because they'd promised to help, and they didn't. I said to myself, *"You know what? Why am I putting myself in this position? I put my faith in someone and was let down. I don't want to be in this position."*

This awakening started from that painful, traumatic moment I felt I was let down, and showed me that I needed to take full responsibility for my finances – so that's exactly what I did the next year. You should be open to the awakening – go towards the pain and not away from it. It turned out to be the biggest gift. You have to accept the pain and surrender to wherever you are in that moment. Look for the insights that come to you. Sometimes you may have to wait for those insights, but they will come.

What if you can't find any awakening or insights?

Listen to that inner voice, and follow what you are curious about. There is indeed a little voice saying something to you – otherwise you wouldn't be here today. You wouldn't be reading this book if you felt you've transformed and have everything you ever wanted in life. You're reading this book because you want answers, and you will get those answers from within. That's why I am here to guide you.

What if the trigger is not in the form of extreme pain? If it's not a major event or trauma, it's a 'nagging' – a curiosity that triggers your interest and wants your attention. What are you curious about? What are you interested in these days? Look into whether that path will lead you to the answer.

What do I do if I feel stuck in the situation I am in?

If you do nothing about where you are right now, nothing will change. You are still stuck in that vicious cycle. You have options, though. It's your life. You can take 100% responsibility for your life, and you decide what to do. You can decide to be negative and disapproving of your situation, or be positive and loving. I decided to be positive and loving, and I got my answers.

What if I think my situation is so different that I can't change it?

Again, it comes down to you. When I feel like this, I decide to get myself into a resourceful state by moving my body – even if it's for a short walk or jumping around and exercising.

The way you're focusing and reading your situation is not accurate because you're upset. There's nothing wrong with you. Take a step back, radically change your physiology, get some energy going, and let the answers come to you. There is a powerful awakening waiting for you.

Activity 1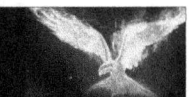

UNLEASH YOUR INNER PHOENIX

Make a list of the top five areas of your life that you are unhappy with.
List them in order, with Priority 1 being the area you are most unhappy with, and so on.
Then consider why this is.

Priority	Areas I am unhappy with	Why?
1.		
2.		
3.		
4.		
5.		

Chapter 4

H for Hyper Inner-Vibe Audit

"Everything in the universe is within you. Ask all from yourself."- Rumi.

A hyper inner-vibe audit is about looking within and really auditing our own thoughts, emotions and feelings. It's about understanding what we're really feeling about the area/s of our life that we've said we are unhappy with (like those in the previous chapter).

I'll never forget that moment I was sitting in my room in June 2019. I realised my life was a mess, and I needed to reflect on everything that had happened to me up until that moment. I didn't know it at the time, but that was the beginning of my hyper inner-vibe audit.

The benefits of doing the audit

This whole thing is about self-discovery, self-awareness and healing all your wounds. You get great insights, and it helps you process what you're going through. You can finally identify your real feelings and release them. You surrender and accept where you are at. After the powerful awakening, this stage is your Audit Stage – which is very important.

Don't go into the next step without completing the activities in this chapter. Nothing will change if you do nothing, and you won't understand why these triggers and events keep happening. You'll also be stuck in a place you don't want to be.

How will you do this audit? What will you do?

First, you need to understand the issue you're experiencing, and why this event/trigger is happening. I suggest you really go deep to understand what is going on. A good start would be to ask yourself the following questions:

- **What do I believe is the issue?**
- **Why is this bothering me?**
- **What is the meaning I have given this event/trigger?**
- **What is the gift in this?**
- **What are the lessons from this?**
- **Why does this happen?**
- **What is the truth in this?**

However, you need to be calm and in a balanced state first. When you're upset, angry and feeling sad, your thinking won't be very clear.

Before you do any of this audit, you must self-soothe first. So, if you broke up with someone or got fired from a job that day, self-soothing could be anything from sitting in bed, feeling like a victim, or just allowing yourself to be sad, angry, hurt or numb, depending on the stress response you had. In the past, I have tried so many things to soothe myself, like listening to sad songs, energy clearing meditations, going for a walk, or even curling up in bed for a day. I've also binge-watched Netflix. That's fine, too. Do something you absolutely love.

If you don't want to do anything, and you want to just curl up in bed and just sleep for the whole day, that's fine, too. Do whatever you need to do. It's whatever you need to do to attain your equilibrium, as you can't go through this process when you are upset. I am not saying for one minute that your feelings are not valid. They are very valid, and that is the reason we are at this step.

However, we need to move through the feelings to access our inner knowing and truth. We do this by accessing universal intelligence, and it's more helpful to be in a balanced and neutral state. I just surrender to my emotions and feelings, and I accept the moment

I am in. I accept the failure and the result, because it is exactly the way it is. You can't change it.

Every thought you have is yours. Therefore, we need to take responsibility for your thinking in order to change. You may not be able to control the event, but you can certainly control your response to it. This inner vibe audit is about learning how to do just that.

Meditation

Another technique that could be useful for this step in the framework is to engage in a meditation practice. Meditation helps us to go beyond the mind and access the higher universal intelligence that will help you find the answers you are looking for.

Meditation does not have to be complicated – there are lots of free apps out there that are easy to access with a Google search. However, I am going to share a really simple process that I follow, and I can do this on my own without any external music or apps:

1. **Sit on the floor or chair with your spine straight.**

2. **Remain still and close your eyes.**

3. **Focus on your normal breath just as an observer.**

4. **Start inhaling through your nose for four counts, then exhale through your mouth for four counts. Do this up to eight times.**

5. **Notice how you are feeling. Observe every part of your body from head to toe, and imagine it relaxing more and more with every breath.**

6. **If any thoughts come up, that's natural. Just observe it like a guest and let it go.**

7. **Do this for at least eighteen minutes a day.**

As soon as you come out of this meditation, complete activity two and three that comes later in this chapter. The idea is that meditation helps you come to a neutral state, which is the best place to find those innermost answers and insights.

What if you don't like the experience of going inward and doing an inner vibe audit?

So you learnt that you don't like going inward. I did an audit when I had that relationship breakdown and it brought up some really uncomfortable feelings and truths that I had to see and accept. It is hard – I get it – however this step is key to help us process our feelings and have meaningful insights to help us move forward.

They say the truth pisses us off at first, but then it sets you free. I am encouraging you to examine your discomfort, then ask yourself why it makes you uncomfortable – what are those feelings pointing to? Really examine those feelings. It's worth doing in the end.

I realised that I don't like being treated in a particular way. I didn't like how I put myself in a situation where that happened, and I realised I didn't set boundaries or do the necessary things to establish a healthy relationship, and that was because of the unhealed past traumas of my last relationship.

Once you've accepted, surrendered and self-soothed, what also really helps is to forgive the person you think is to blame for this situation. That person could be you, so you must forgive yourself. You don't have to make the other person right or wrong. Neither do you have to agree with them. You don't have to love them or anything. You just have to understand why this is happening and why you are responding the way you are.

By forgiving, you can begin the healing process. You'll probably find that it's not even the person you're angry with – it's probably linked to something that's happened in your childhood. The events that trigger us are gifts that help us see where the wounds are, so that we can heal them.

As humans, we either have a fight, flight or freeze response to an event that scares or triggers us. I become so overwhelmed that I usually have a freeze response where I become paralysed, and I can't do anything about it. I'm finding, though, that I just must let myself surrender to that moment. I just do what I can, and I start to feel a bit better once the nerves calm down. I can go through the actual audit, release those emotions, identify what they are, take responsibility for them and process them.

For forgiveness particularly, when it comes to relationships, I use the Hawaiian practice called ho'oponopono, from a course I did, and I really love it. It is pretty straightforward. You can think about the person you are angry or upset with, and say:

- **I am sorry.**
- **I love you.**
- **I forgive you.**
- **Thank you.**

If you feel it's your fault, you can think about the person you feel you hurt and say:

- **Can you please forgive me?**
- **I'm sorry.**
- **I love you.**
- **Thank you.**

If you keep that as your intention and keep going, it will help you come back to some sort of equilibrium. Then you can dive in. If you still have those disapproving and negative feelings within you, you won't be able to get clear and work through the audit process. This will help you to clarify what you want.

You can use this forgiveness process to forgive yourself as well if you feel you could have done better in certain times in your life in areas of work, health or friends. After all, we must learn to be kind and compassionate towards our selves first.

What did you realise about yourself and your current results in life?

You can do the inner vibe audit in different areas of your life. Use the answers from Activity 1 in the previous chapter to map out where you currently are in each area of your life – your family life, career, health, wealth, finances, business, social and spiritual goals. This way you can try to understand what is really going on with you. It also helps you objectively acknowledge the situation that has triggered you, and what has happened. I realised I wasn't providing myself with the correct nutrition, but when I did WILDFIT I learnt so much about nutrition and what is good for me.

Those are some of the lessons you learn as part of the program – but you can only learn this once you process the heavy emotions you're dealing with. This is all part of this hyper inner vibe audit. It's about to get really clear. It's about acknowledging, *"So this is my current state. This is where I am."*

I've always believed that working on your health first is essential before you tackle everything else. After all, health is wealth. If you don't have your health, it's all just a pipe dream. In my case, it's always helped to keep health as my number one priority. I also applied the P.H.O.E.N.I.X. Framework in my financial life and relationships, and made some significant shifts in these areas.

What is it you want? If you don't want it this way, how does it need to change?

Once you have mapped out where you currently are in each area of your life, the next part of this audit process is to get really clear on what you want so you can manifest it in your life.

Activity 2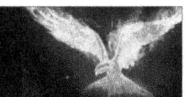

Take your priority 1 area from our last activity and answer the following questions in a reflective, quiet environment. Repeat for each of the top priority areas.

Area I am unhappy with	
What is the gift in this?	
What are the lessons?	
Why does this happen?	
What is the truth in this?	

If you're upset about trying to make changes with your finances and not getting anywhere, make a list of what is important to you in that aspect. Write down three essential goals around that area. You can't learn from it if you don't have self-awareness.

There's nothing like failure in life. There are only opportunities to learn something new so you can do things differently. If you don't do this work and the reflection, you won't get these valuable insights. I did the reflection, and I realised I wasn't pleased with my body and health. I realised I wasn't confident around people, and I was frustrated. I came out of this exercise with a Hyper Inner Vibe Audit, and I would not have been able to do it if I had not really tuned in.

Even now, I am only sharing my experience of how *I* did it. This is my experience of the framework. I don't know the answers to all your problems, but you might get your answers faster if you go through the steps in this framework. I've made mistakes, and I've done a lot of work around this. I've done my own personal development for over ten years. I work with many coaches, and that's why I've realised that this step is crucial as part of your transformation journey. Don't shy away from it.

I have learnt many lessons, and I am sharing them with you here so that you can learn from them, too, and save time.

What if you feel you have no control over the events that happen in your life?

Say you have an injury that's preventing you from exercising, or you didn't get the job you wanted because COVID hit and you could not get to your interview in time. Again, you have to surrender and accept things the way they are.

You also have to take full ownership of your life – if you don't, you're putting the power in someone else's hands. That's not what you want. Ask yourself what went wrong, then decide what you would do differently next time.

The reason this is useful is that you can never change an external event or how another person behaves. You can only change your own behaviour and attitude.

Activity 3

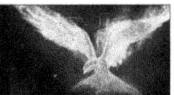

List of things you believe were mistakes, what you learnt from it and what you would do differently next time.

My top five mistakes I believe I have made	What I learnt from it	What I would do differently next time
1.		
2.		
3.		
4.		
5.		

You are an adult – you decide how you want to lead your life and what you want to get out of it. Rejection is part of life. Sometimes you don't get the job you want, even though you were a solid candidate. You could fall pregnant after years of trying, only to have a miscarriage – or the person you thought things would work out with didn't feel the same way about you. Your life is nobody else's responsibility but yours. All that people owe you is basic human decency and respect – they don't owe you love or money. I know that sounds harsh, but that is the truth.

It's time for you to take responsibility and do the audit of your own life. Is your inner vibe high or low? If you have a low vibe, you'll feel unhappy, anxious, stagnant or stuck, and worry you won't get to where you want to be. You want to get to a high vibe, where you feel alive and inspired to take action. You'll feel clear on your purpose and why you want to do something. It's okay to start where you are. Good luck.

Activity 4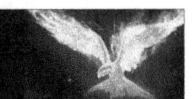

UNLEASH YOUR INNER PHOENIX

For each of the top five priority areas in your life, write up to three goals in each area that will make you feel happy and give you a sense of achievement.

Priority	Areas I am unhappy with	Why?	Three goals in each area that will make me happy when they happen.
1.			• • •
2.			• • •
3.			• • •
4.			• • •
5.			• • •

Chapter 5

O for Open New Pathways

"You were born with wings, so why crawl through life?"- Rumi.

Once you're clear on what areas you want to focus on in your life, you begin to see pathways open for you in ways that you have never observed before. This may be because you were not clear and focused on what you really wanted.

Once you are clear on your plans and intentions by doing your full inner vibe audit, you will find out which areas you're unhappy with. I would suggest you look at these.

When I was doing my inner audit, I sat in my room and realised why my life was failing in many aspects. I basically decided to focus on three things. The main one was health, finances and then I also had another focus on my lack of social connection.

I found I was lacking social connection and feeling quite lonely. Many of my school and university friends were overseas, and my friends in Australia were married and had their own lives. I was really looking to build a supportive community around me – one that suited the healthy lifestyle I was working towards, and a community I could be myself around. I wanted to improve my social capital – so I started looking out for some supportive communities to belong to.

The second aspect I focused on was finance. I shifted my focus here because I felt I needed to get my finances sorted if I really wanted to do things the way I wanted.

Then of course I also focused on my health.

Finding a role model

I decided that the best way for me to approach all these things was to have a role model. Your mind is like a map, but you need know where to go. I found WILDFIT for my health transformation, and I wanted to find some equivalent role models who were doing well in the community and the finance spaces.

Role models are the people who've been through the journey and made all the mistakes. In the end, they found a way through it and are willing to share that information with you, show you a shortcut as to how it's done. I would certainly suggest you investigate finding the right role model for you and your goals.

Find someone you resonate with, look up to and someone who inspires you. You must find someone who could be that role model for you, then start spending a lot more time engaging with them, either via their online platform or through a one-on-one meeting. Obviously, the person who you approach must also be open and invested in coaching you.

Sometimes you don't need to approach them directly – they may be offering an online workshop, or a product you can purchase or subscribe to that can help you (for example, how I did the online WILDFIT 90-day Challenge program). People want to share and help because they feel it is their purpose, which is why I am doing this. I feel it's my purpose to share this message with you because I've had this experience and know it works.

On this journey, I will give you the tools and things you might find helpful, but you need to be clear about what you want. Get clear on what you want, then look for someone who can help you with the information that can get you there.

Setting your goals

I hope you realise that even someone like me, who's been through all the crap life threw at me, can get my shit together. If I can go for it, why can't you? I am not saying I'm there 100%. I am a little ahead of the journey than you are, and that's why I can show you what

I did. It's my experience, but many people are role models in the areas I learned from, so there's always someone who can help. Therefore, you need to be clear on what you want, find those role models, invest time in listening and engaging with them, and immerse yourself in the knowledge they have to offer.

It's helpful to do visualisation practices. Visualisation is a process where we imagine what we want to happen in our lives and see it in our minds like it has already happened. When we visualize, we make it possible for these images to come alive in reality. There are heaps of free content for visualisations and meditations available on SoundCloud, Spotify and YouTube.

What happens once you set these goals?

You become a magnet to these goals once you get clear. You will see opportunities and coincidences show up because you're clear, and it will feel like magic.

When I was agitated, I realised that I wanted to work on my health, and I was looking for a role model to help me with that. I stumbled upon WILDFIT, and at that point I knew I was ready. The moment the teacher showed up, my life was completely changed. WILDFIT completely altered my health. I'd been told I had a hormonal imbalance and polycystic ovarian syndrome. Through WILDFIT, I learnt about proper nutrition so that I could tackle these health concerns.

What if I don't find my role model?

You will when you are clear. I am also sure you're not one of those people who won't take action. If you follow this framework every time you have things come up, you'll reach your goal.

What if I feel it is too much change?

Change is constant, and transformation is eternal, which is why the phoenix is so powerful. The phoenix keeps dying into ashes, then reincarnates itself from those ashes – which will also happen to us several times in this lifetime.

If you feel it's too much change and you can't do it on your own, you should rally your own support, mentors and people around you. Find your community. For my health goals, I am involved in the WILDFIT Community. I engaged in challenges with my peers. We have an amazing private Facebook group, and a fantastic peer group – the WILDFIT Coaches Community.

I found a great dance and wellbeing community for my social goals. I found an amazing group which hosts regular get-togethers with a lot of wellness components included, like exercise and yoga. These get-togethers are generally sober events with no alcohol involved. The group also hosts music healing sessions, which are second to none. The people I met there have become amazing friends.

I highly recommend joining communities because it opens new pathways. Just by doing WILDFIT, I met so many amazing people, and I've even decided to start my own business. I now have an amazing community of coaches.

Picking yourself back up

As humans, we will always have shit days. When you have these shit days, what you need is a supportive network to say, *"Hey, you're not all bad. You're not crap. You're beating yourself up too much."*

Nobody's perfect, and nobody's got all the answers. We all need help sometimes. If we work collaboratively, one of us will have the answer, and that's the idea. Community is immunity. Even now when I have off days, and I realise I'm not following the plan, I call my community coach and let them know what's happening. They help me work through it. Even coaches need coaches.

What if I can't afford to spend money on courses and mentors?

You don't need to spend a lot of money. Thanks to YouTube, there are a lot of free resources available out there. I found these gave me a lot of value and helped me out. Subsequently I did several paid courses that other business leaders offer. You've got to start where you are.

You have to remember the journey that has brought you here. You have to remember what you went through. We all went through the pain, then we had the powerful awakening. We basically said, *"Oh my God, the universe is trying to get my attention. I need to listen to these messages, and I need to do my Inner Vibe Audit. I got really clear on what I need to do. Now, I am trying to find new ways to achieve that result."*

Can you afford not to do the inner audit work, considering where you're coming from?

This is an opportunity to step up, to get to the next step. This is the opportunity for you to really get some support to get your goals and open new pathways.

You should remember your purpose. Go back to it, and you will find a way and get results. You should always put a positive twist on your emotions and say, *"What are the opportunities here?"*

Activity 5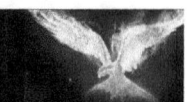

I strongly encourage you to write down your goals around the areas you feel you're not happy with, then find role models who are doing really well in those areas.
Research what content they are offering that is available on the internet or via presentations.

Areas I am unhappy with	Who do I know/respect in this area who could be my role model?	What about them do I admire?	What courses/books/free content do they have to offer?
1.			
2.			
3.			
4.			
5.			

Chapter 6

E for Energy Rising

"As you start to walk out on the way, the way appears." - Rumi.

"Energy Rising" is all about gaining momentum and going all in with your goals. After you are clear on what you want and you've got the help from all your role models, you know that you're invested. You can then decide to go ahead and follow your role model's suggestions.

You need to go all in. You have to give yourself a chance to let your energy rise from within, and the only way you'll do that is by fully committing and embracing the process. You need to be wholly committed as that's the only way you will get your results.

The process needs to be fully immersive. You need to implement what happens practically. As you go, you'll get more engaged and find more motivation to keep going. You'll find that your energy will rise, you will get momentum and you'll feel better about yourself and what you can do. That is everything. That is the step of the journey that is really critical.

Sometimes, you won't like some of the stuff you have to do, but you just have to keep doing it to get the result. Not giving up on those things will make you grow, and your goals will be met. It will also enrich your life experiences.

Don't wait for the motivation. Do it first, then the motivation will come. That's what you need to do. If you don't do it all, nothing will change and you'll still be in the same place.

You haven't embraced the process. You've done all the work, but what you have is only intellectual knowledge and you don't know how to use it.

Commit to change

To be successful, the first thing you need to do is show up, then commit to putting in the work. If you don't show up, you won't get the results you need because you have not taken the first step towards the goal.

You need to make a decision to commit to the process. The pain I felt before I had my awakening was so raw, and after my audit, I was really clear about my purpose. I found my mentors, and all that was left was for me to make a decision, commit entirely and go for it. There is no turning back. You have to stay committed. However, you can stay flexible in your approach. You need to have a plan of where you need to get to. You may have setbacks, and you might have to adapt a little bit on the way. As long as you're moving in the right direction, it's okay.

Get organised. Schedule and plan things. If it's not in the calendar, it won't happen. It's just like when I decided to do WILDFIT, I registered and put my credit card down. I registered for the course, and that was it. I knew I was committed. I knew I was in when I made that decision.

Shake the fear

Just before you decide, observe the thoughts that you have – because that's where the fear shows up. Fear may cause you to feel you don't want to do it at all. You might tell yourself a hundred reasons why you shouldn't do it. Your inner critic says, *"What is going to be different about this one? It's all going to be the same."*

That's when you need to stick to your guns. The only way things are going to happen is if you make plans, schedule it, make the payment, book that meeting, call that person, send that text message and take action. You have to be in it for the long-term – and for long-term change and permanent transformation, you need to be consistent. Consistency trumps talent – so even if you were born talented, if you don't practice and be consistent about getting better, you won't achieve your goals. If you are consistent, you will get your results because you are practicing. That keeps you on track.

I can give you an example that comes up with this. When I was doing WILDFIT, I needed to take a break from certain things I felt I couldn't live without. When I gave these up, I had a massive headache the first few days and experienced massive withdrawal symptoms. I felt nauseous and in so much pain, but I still showed up to every WILDFIT video that was sent to me. I showed up to every coaching call I had.

By the end of that particular week, I was wowed. These were things I thought I could never give up, but I'd given them up. I've demonstrated to myself that believing that I couldn't give them up was bullshit, because I did it after three days of headache, and I felt amazing.

"What are the other things I've been telling myself are impossible?" I wondered. *"If I can do this, what else can I do?"* That's the place you want to get to, and the momentum you want to gain. You show up. Stick to the process and you'll find your energy rising and your self-esteem building. You'll be surprised at what you can achieve!

Make the time

When I was becoming a coach, some of the personal development courses and training I had to attend were held in US time, which means it was always night time here in Australia. After quite a few all-nighters, I would still work during the day. I had not slept, and I still showed up to the live class.

I once did a personal development program that had me stay up three whole nights, and I did it because I wanted to show up and be engaged. I've done many WILDFIT Mastermind calls by staying up at 2am and 3am, and I still had to go to work the next morning. The reason I did this is because when you show up live, you are telling the universe, *"I'm freaking serious about this. This is something I want to do. This means something to me."*

If you're in a situation where you can't show up for the live session, that's fine. Sometimes there are replays for the course videos. But when you show up live, you're engaging with a live audience, and there's more accountability. In live sessions, there are more peer group interactions. You basically become more engaged, and you get more immersed when you are more engaged. The course content and transformation is more internalised, and you get a result.

When you come to a moment of truth, you know you need to make a decision to do something. If you are unsure about what decision to make, perhaps you need to go back to the earlier steps to see why you're not making these decisions.

What is stopping me?

It is most probably fear. Deal with the fear, release the fear, and deal with what is happening. Make a decision, then take action. When you make a proper decision, you decide that there's nothing to look back on. Once you make a decision, you begin to feel good about it and move forward. That's the amount of commitment you need.

When you do this, you find that your energy rises. That's building your self-esteem up as well. You have taken your first step out of a hard situation. You decided to take up the call. Sometimes, you don't have to see the whole summit or know how to climb it. You will get to the summit, but you just need to take one step after the other and be consistent about it.

You know what? If you fail in your path, that's usually due to your fear. Don't beat yourself up – just get back up and get back into the game. Your mindset plays a critical role, then you go back to examine your purpose. *Why am I doing this? Why have I decided?* Then you remember the pain and make this your drive to succeed. *I've done the inner audit. I have a different vision for my life right now. I need to go forward*. Those are the things that will give you momentum.

You might be wondering what happens if you lose interest. Always remember your purpose, as it replenishes your energy. You need to go back to why you're here. *Why am I in this situation?*

Look how far you've come and what you have achieved so far. Don't just focus on how far away you are from your goal, but also think about your progress so far. That will give you enough energy to rise to the next level, which comprises all you want and desire in life.

Activity 6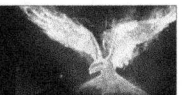

UNLEASH YOUR INNER PHOENIX

Identify any potential fears/resistance that might be stopping you for moving forward and immersing yourself in the journey.

Areas I am unhappy with	What are my fears around achieving the goals around this area?	What is my resistance towards having the goals in this area?	Where have I failed in this area before?	What is the next best step I can take to move forward with the goals in this area?
1.				
2.				
3.				
4.				
5.				

Chapter 7

N for Not Giving Up

"When everything seems to oppose you, when you feel you cannot even bear one more minute, never give up – because it is the time and place that the course will divert."
- Rumi.

"Not giving up" is exactly what it says. At this stage of the framework, we have to keep going no matter what, and not give up on everything we have done so far. I know you're tired, but keep going because it's very important. You have come this far, and you're very close to the summit.

You want to do this because it will boost your self-pride. You will appreciate yourself more by knowing how far you've come, and you will completely transform from within, which is what this whole journey is about. You will get the desired results, and they will be noticeable. So many people go through life without fulfilling their dreams because they gave up too soon. You don't want to be one of those people. Many people on their deathbeds express regret that they gave up on the things that mattered most.

There is always a way. You have to change your approach at times because you will encounter things that won't work. As I said before, as long as you know where you're going and the outcome you want, you can adapt your approach to achieve your goals – but giving up is not an option. Giving up will attract nothing but regret, and regret is worse than any feeling of failure that you can have.

According to Thomas Edison, the three greatest things that are essential in life are 'hard work, stick-to-itiveness and common sense.' Stick-to-itiveness is essential because that's the premise of this chapter. Keep going until you get achieve your goal. Don't stop.

Of course, there will be obstacles. Of course it's going to get hard. Nobody said it is going to be easy. Remember, this is the P.H.O.E.N.I.X. Framework. This is where you let go of your old habits, old beliefs and old patterns because they're clearly not working for you. We need to do something different to get a different result.

So, how do you deal with the failure?

Of course, you can hit obstacles. You have to expect them. I can give you an example of a WILDFIT client of mine who was doing great on the challenge till she tripped on the stairs in her apartment and broke her ankle. This required surgery and six weeks off her feet. I would have understood if she'd wanted to give up, but she didn't – she had a supportive husband who cooked for her and helped her stay on track. She even joined the WILDFIT coaching calls when she was not at the physio, and listened to the recording later.

This journey requires you to become a leader. A leader will want to keep going and never give up. A leader will lead, not follow. A leader will defy all the odds and set new standards to achieve goals. You need to anticipate any mistakes that may happen and correct them as you go. If the old plan didn't work, change it and make a new one. Find another way.

There's always a way, and you can get back on track after failure. If you fall ten times, get back up the eleventh time and keep going. After getting up, use a different approach, and never make the same mistakes.

Go back to your mentors. This is where the community, your support network and your role model come in. That's how you can get advice on how to get the results.

How can you recover from failing?

How can you handle the fear, rejection and resistance? How can you observe your self-talk and correct it? What you want is to know how to cope. Pick yourself up, dust yourself off and have another go.

All these things will keep you on track. Of course, your purpose is always important. You have to know what you want your outcome to be, and why you're following your purpose. You're doing it because you experienced a significant amount of emotional discomfort. You weren't happy where you were. Then you got clear and decided on what you want.

You need to keep going. You're at the stage where you are close to achieving your results because you've done all the work. You've come so far in your journey. Look at how far you've come, not at how far you have to go. It will be a shame if you give up at this point as you're so close.

My WILDFIT Coaching Journey

Let me share the story of my WILDFIT coaching journey. It was a six-month journey, very comprehensive, and yes, I showed up for all the classes. If I wasn't able to make it, I was listening to the replays. I got up at 4am or 5am for at least twelve weeks because I had to have live engagements with the Master Coaches. I asked great questions, immersed myself in the process, and did all the things I'm telling you guys to do.

The first step was to do a written exam, which I prepared for and completed. The second stage was completing the course material again, and then the third stage was the trial class. This was where most coaches fall off track. Our Master Coaches told us this upfront, so we knew we should expect some difficulties and obstacles around this part of the journey.

Just when it was time for me to do my trial classes, COVID-19 hit. In the middle of the pandemic, many people thought it wasn't possible to do anything productive, but here I was, trying to launch and start a new business. I was also trying to get a coaching certification and trying to tell people to get healthy. I believed there was no better time to get a healthy immune system. Health is everything and that message was really clear, especially in the new pandemic world we're living in. But I was struggling to get a group together to give this trial class a go. I was getting a lot of support and other people were happy for me, but I couldn't convince anybody to actually do the trial class with me.

I was almost going to give up. I said to myself, *"Why am I trying to do this on top of what was going on, at a time when the whole world is going through a pandemic? This is crazy. I don't want to do this. Maybe I should just give up."*

I asked a few people to join the trial classes, but they were just not ready. Now I know you can't get people to do it unless they're actually ready – but at the time I took it personally, as people who told me they were going to the trial classes backed out, and I felt I wasn't getting any support. I didn't know how I could do this with the whole world in lockdown.

Then I just made up my mind and said, *"You know what? Why am I doing this? I am becoming a coach because WILDFIT works, and I have had a personal transformation.*

This message is crucial to share, and I need to complete my certification. I've invested my hard-earned money in it. I have to find a way."

I got a few of my closest friends together and said, "Guys, you need to support me." Then I did what I needed to do and got a very small group together. I set a date and set up my new class. I didn't care about how big or small it was. I had enough people to help, and I decided I would just go for it. I am so glad I did because the trial class results were so overwhelmingly positive for my clients. On hearing the positive results, I realised how purposeful I was. The moral of the story is to never give up.

Getting back up again

I can share another example where I was supposed to take a break from alcohol, but I went out one weekend with my friends and had two glasses of tequila. I felt sick afterwards, and I wondered why I'd done it. I'd ruined everything. I'd failed. I was five weeks into the challenge, and I'd been going so well. I had given up and was really beating myself up.

Then I decided not to let that slip up make me feel like I was a failure. I had to get back on track again. I went back to the community and peer group I was doing my challenge with and said, "Hey guys, I need support here." It's about asking for help and support. I wasn't really good at doing that, but now I've become better at it. When you are vulnerable and ask for help, many people are waiting and willing. You just need to ask the right people. You can also ask the people who have earned your trust to do that.

After meeting with my community, I was back on track. I was back into the WILDFIT Challenge, and I completed the challenge without any hitches.

Learning to push forward

In your challenge or journey, there's always a point you will encounter difficulties. That is not the time to give up. It is the time to press the accelerator up and go forward. That is what I've learnt from my experience.

The same thing happened with my corporate career. Years ago, I was in the leading branch in one of the largest top four banks in Australia, and I was a middle management leader. They were very good to me. I went for a leadership course, and I decided that it was time for me to change my career.

I went ahead and pursued what I was really good at – connecting with people. Luckily, I connected with the right person who needed to help me as a role model. She was an expert in what I wanted to do, which was organisational change. I connected with her and asked if she could be my mentor. She said she could, but she was very time poor and I had to follow up quite a few times. There was a time that we were supposed to meet, but she declined the meeting. Although she was apologetic, it just wasn't working out.

I was trying to connect with different people, but I just wasn't getting anywhere. I then decided to do what was in my control. I would focus on what I could to do my job really well. At that point, I just surrendered and accepted where I was. Out of the blue, my mentor gave me a call and said she'd just had a conversation with someone about interviewing, and I got my breakthrough. I was able to push through and make a change in my career.

I think that's been a very instrumental part of success in my career and professional life. I feel the skills I acquired through this organisational and personal change gave me the credibility to write this book. This is because I've seen how change works at a personal level.

The program will work if you just stick to your guns. You need to find a way to stay in the game. The only game you can play is the game in front of you. However, if the game is not in your favour, find a different approach and keep your eyes on the next game.

What if you feel if your goals are not in your control?

If you have the right connections, people, knowledge and dedication, you won't have any problem reaching your goals. All you need to do is handle your part and show up. If you don't do your part, nobody else will do that on your behalf.

You should also know it's okay to be rejected. It shouldn't make you feel less human. Therefore, you need to get used to being rejected. People are telling you what they actually want. The only thing people owe you is human decency and respect. If you have that, it's okay.

In the case of rejection, find another person who can help you with your goal. You can always find another way to get your desired results. Never give up on yourself and your goals.

Activity 7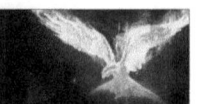

Use this activity to list the times that you pushed through your feelings of wanting to give up, only to use these feelings to give you some momentum. Get clear on what's stopping you from achieving your goal. You can't make a plan to achieve your goal if you are not clear on what the issue is.

List some examples of a time you wanted to give up but kept going. What was the result?	
List how you have handled the fear, rejection and resistance that has come up in the past when you were striving for a goal	
For the goal you are currently working on, list any failings, circumstances, reasons or excuses that are coming up for you to give up on the goal	
Observe your self-talk and list it down. Is it caused by fear or resistance to the issue?	
Who can you reach out to who can help you find a solution to progress this goal?	

Chapter 8

I for 'I am at the Next Level'

"Stop acting so small. You are the universe in ecstatic motion." - Rumi.

You have reached a milestone in your journey. Now it's time to acknowledge that and celebrate the progress you have made so far. This is when you start to see results after starting your journey. You will feel like a whole new person and feel more creative because the changes are visible.

When I was working on my health, my weight loss was evident, and people noticed that I had a natural glow more energy. My skin was glowing, but more importantly it was all about inner confidence – that inner belief that you can achieve anything that you want.

If you can do this, what else can you do?

That's the kind of strong foundation you set every time you do something transformational. In fact, you should be congratulating yourself for going through all that discomfort during the process. You showed up, showed commitment and made decisions.

Now is the time you set yourself up to get to the next level. You need to celebrate the results you have got. If you decide that this is too painful to embrace, you won't leave your comfort zone and do what is necessary to get the results. You will find it difficult or impossible to achieve the desired results. This is also about the time that people will start noticing and complimenting you because you now have a completely new lease on life. They may ask you how you did it.

You have complete creativity and discovery of what's possible. You now feel more connected and as though many things are possible. This is all about celebrating where you are, and getting closer to your goal.

Discovering a new part of you

You are a spiritual being. You are on a spiritual journey in a human form. This shows you that you can be a better version of yourself. The Phoenix is rising as part of this transformation.

What I found was that I started hanging out with communities that were supportive of my new food habits. I was very comfortable making a healthy choice at dinner if I caught up with my other friends. More importantly, I discovered a completely different arena for food.

I stopped shopping in the same place I used to. I set myself to a higher standard, and I went for it. For instance, I would look at recipes and change the ingredients I knew were not good for me. I changed some of these recipes because I noticed my body's reaction to them, and I had to choose healthier options. As a result, I started becoming more passionate about cooking, and I decided to share many of my food pictures on Instagram.

I am not a perfect cook. I did not do any culinary studies, but I was just so excited when I saw people's engagements after they saw my food pictures on Instagram. They would ask me for the recipe, and I would readily share them because I really wanted to inspire people to make better food choices.

Here are a few of my go-tos that use WILDFIT-friendly ingredients!

Tuna Steak with Fresh Salsa

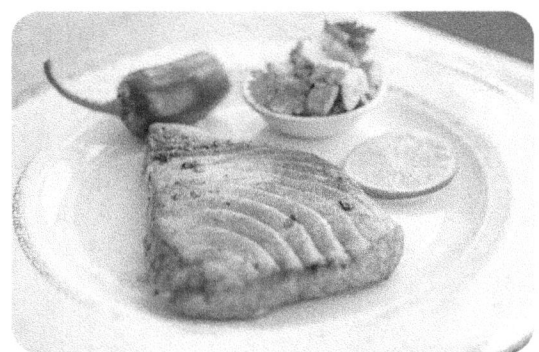

Details

Prep time: 24 mins
Cook time: 6 mins
Total time: 30 mins

Ingredients

For Fish

- 1 tuna steak (ideally wild caught or organic)
- 2 tbsp olive oil
- ¼ tsp smoky paprika
- ¼ tsp red chilli flakes
- ¼ tsp pepper
- ¼ tsp salt or to taste
- ¼ lemon

For Salsa

- 3 tbsp extra virgin oil
- 1 small avocado
- ¼ red onion, chopped fine
- 4 cherry tomatoes, chopped
- ¼ jalapeno chilli
- ¼ tsp pepper
- ¼ tsp salt or to taste
- ¼ lime
- Small handful of chopped coriander leaves

Instructions

1. Marinate the fish in a bowl with 1 tbsp oil, and all the spices that have been combined into a paste, for at least for 15 minutes.
2. In a non-stick fry pan, add the remaining oil and heat for 30 seconds.
3. Add fish and shallow fry for 2-3 minutes each side or until cooked.
4. Combine all chopped veggies in the olive oil, except coriander leaves and lime.
5. Once combined, taste for salt and squeeze in lime. Garnish with coriander leaves.
6. Serve with tuna steak on the side and enjoy!

South Indian Blue Swimmer Crab Stir Fry

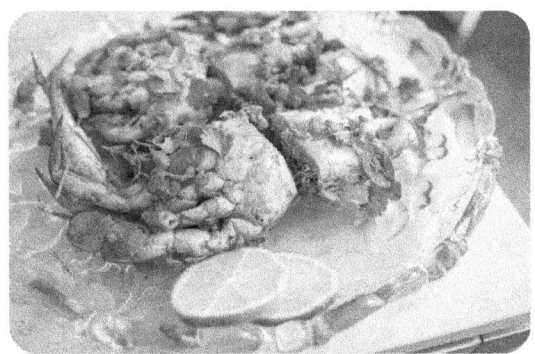

Details

Prep time: 20 minutes
Cook time: 15 mins
Total time: 35 mins

Ingredients

- 2 blue swimmer crabs (or any crab), cleaned and cut into pieces
- 4 tbsp coconut/olive oil
- 1 medium onion
- 6 cherry tomatoes
- 2 cloves of garlic
- 4-5 curry leaves
- ½ inch fresh ginger thinly sliced
- ½ tsp black mustard seeds
- ¼ tsp turmeric
- ¼ tsp chilli powder or red chilli flakes
- ¼ tsp pepper
- ¼ tsp salt or to taste
- Small bunch of coriander leaves for garnish
- 1 lime, sliced

Instructions

1. In a non-stick pan, add mustard seeds, curry leaves, chopped onion, garlic and ginger in the oil that's been heated for 30 seconds.
2. Stir fry for at least 3-4 minutes until the onions turn golden brown.
3. Add the dry spices and combine for stir fry for another minute or so.
4. Add the crab and combine with the masala. Make sure every part of the crab has been coated.
5. Cover the pan and let the crab steam in the juices in the base. There should be enough water coming out of the crab – if not, add a couple of tsp of water.
6. When crab is cooked, serve and garnish with lime slices and coriander leaves.

Healthy Ferrero Rocher Balls

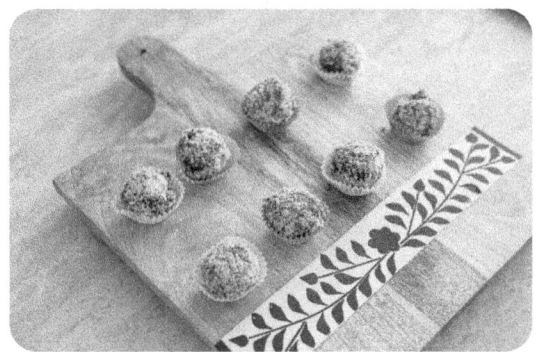

Details

Prep time: 10 mins
Cook time: No cook
Total time: 20 mins

Ingredients

- 1 cup medjool dates, pitted
- ½ cup hazelnuts
- 2 teaspoons cacao powder
- ¼ tsp salt
- ½ cup chopped roasted hazelnuts for rolling
- ½ cup whole hazelnuts for the middle of the ball
- ¼ cup organic non-dairy dark chocolate, melted (if you want to avoid chocolate, just roll in with chopped roasted hazelnuts)

Instructions

1. Place dates, cacao, salt and hazelnuts into a food processor or blender. Pulse until combined like a dough.
2. Place a whole hazelnut into the middle, then roll into equal sized balls.
3. Dunk half the ball into the dark chocolate and roll in chopped hazelnuts.
4. Place in the freezer for ten minutes to set. Enjoy!

Delicious Banana Muffins

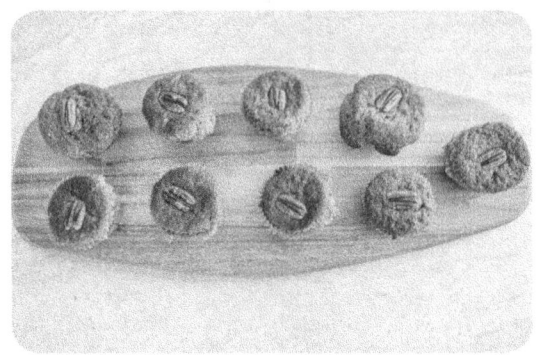

Details

Prep time: 20 minutes
Cook time: 30 minutes
Total time: 50 mins

Ingredients

- 3 ripe bananas (with 1 fresh banana for the top)
- 2 cups almond flour
- ½ cup tapioca flour
- 1 tsp ground cinnamon
- ¼ tsp salt
- 2 eggs
- ¼ cup coconut oil
- ¼ cup? Tsp? honey
- 1 tsp vanilla extract

Instructions

1. Preheat oven to 180°C.
2. Grease the muffin cups with coconut oil and place them in the muffin tray.
3. Mash the three ripe bananas in a mixing bowl. Add remaining ingredients and hand blend or use hand mixer till you have a consistent batter.
4. Pour the batter into each of the muffin cups until full.
5. Slice the fresh banana into small pieces and place on top of each muffin.
6. Place in oven and bake for 25-30 minutes or until baked through.
7. Keep covered with aluminum foil to avoid it becoming too golden.
8. Once baked, let it cool for a few minutes and enjoy!

After changing my diet, I felt like a brand new person from the inside, and I felt I could do anything. That's what you want. I had increased energy. I appreciated the whole journey, and as a result, I appreciated the person I was becoming. I couldn't have done it without a peer group. At this stage, I recommend:

- **Enjoying the journey.**

- **Taking a moment to celebrate and enjoy every little win.**

- **Making a list of all the gains you've had in your journey so far.**

We should be doing this right through the process. The human mind can just as easily focus on what is not going well, but it is more important than ever to pat yourself on the back. Give yourself a high five, then acknowledge the person you've become – because this is you at the next level.

We just need to take the time to look at what we have achieved at this level. For example, there were things I gave up during the challenge that I've never really gone back to. This really was a permanent change as a result of going through that health transformation. That's what most people want. We have all tried yo-yo diets and didn't get the result that we wanted, but with WILDFIT I noticed I was becoming a completely different person.

To embody that behaviour, you need to keep doing things that will keep that behaviour going. For example, start shopping in new places where you can get healthy food. I shop in organic stores for lean meats and organic fruits and vegetables because that's good for me.

I also started cooking a lot more at home and trying out new recipes, which I would never do before. When I was growing up, I was very fond of cooking. I used to cook for my family as my mum travelled a lot, and my little brother enjoyed my food. He would relish what I cooked for him, but I lost that love for cooking over the years as I started working full-time. I had a horrible habit of eating out a lot. There's nothing wrong with eating out with friends, but I was doing it too often, and I just wasn't even enjoying the meal that much.

With this transformation reaching the next level, it reminded me of who I was and the things I used to like to do. Then I regained that love for cooking. This time around, the change was that I was cooking things that were nourishing and good for me. I think that's been one of the biggest wins.

Now when I eat out, another habit I've cultivated is to ask what's in the food I'm eating. I mean, these things are crucial to my health. I would never have done that before WILDFIT – the old me would have never done that. I guess learning has a lot to do with embracing the person you're becoming.

Importance of the right environment around you

When you get to the next level, congratulate yourself and appreciate everything you've done so far. Start hanging out in supportive environments that will support your new behaviours.

There's also more accountability when you are in a similar peer group or community following similar beliefs. When you transform and reach the next level of who you're meant to be, if you don't continue spending time in that tribe or community, you could end up going back to past behaviours. For example, if I was not part of the WILDFIT group, I might go back to old ways and eat things that are not good for me. You need to think about how you want your transformation to be sustainable and embedded in your behaviour permanently.

What if you fail and you don't feel anything different?

If you've taken all the previous steps, you will get the outcome that you want. If you feel you're reverting to your past behaviours, what you need to do is remember why you did the exercise in the first place.

Remember what got you started, and the pain that drove you to do that inner vibe audit. You basically made a plan and found role models, communities and teachers who could help you get there. You did the work and stayed committed to the journey. You now know it's time to start getting results.

Why would you want to go back again? Look back and see how far you have come. You'll then realise you have the leverage to feel like you've got the desired results. There's a reason you've been through this experience, and millions of people would die to know how you did it. You need to step up and be a leader for what you've done. You need to give yourself credit for doing the work. This is next-level stuff.

I for 'I am at the Next Level'

 # Activity 8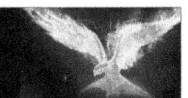

Make a list of all wins, gains and progress you've made for each of your priority areas of focus.

Areas of focus	Wins/Progress/Gain achieved to date
	• • •
	• • •
	• • •
	• • •

Chapter 9

X for Xtra Acceleration

"A heart filled with love is like a phoenix that no cage can imprison." - Rumi.

"Xtra Acceleration" is about celebrating the success you've achieved in your personal transformation journey. These rituals help us recognise how far we have come on our journey and give us inspiration to keep going. This is the time we do everything to really celebrate our success.

You'll feel amazing because this is where the phase of transformation is complete. You feel pretty good about yourself, and you can use this opportunity to reward yourself. Give yourself a treat. (That's actually good for you.)

You'll get to share some of your learnings. This is when you basically want to stay connected to your community because that's the only way you keep learning. After all, proximity is power. You want to continue to re-enforce that learning. When you share what you've learned with others, you're relearn it again. It really helps.

You need to get a look at how you can share what you've learnt and teach someone else what you've done. That way, you are teaching yourself again. If you don't keep doing that, you might find yourself going back to your old behaviours. You definitely don't want that – you've come too far and done so well. Remember, as Zig Ziglar put it, 'Repetition is the mother of learning and the father of action.'

Celebrating your wins

When I reached this stage, I shared my wins with others. In the twelfth week of the 90-Day Challenge, when my trial class was finishing, we had a virtual graduation party to celebrate our successes, and we took it to the next level with Xtra Acceleration. We had a tea ceremony – everyone made a WILDFIT-approved meal and had a beautiful cup of tea. We all got dressed up, took photos of each other and chatted about our experiences and how everyone felt. Sharing how you feel is really important, because it's about that extra acceleration to help you transform completely.

You should also praise other people in your community. Encourage others to keep going. Treat yourself well, and celebrate the moment. Don't be an amateur at this – be a professional at whatever you do.

When I started thinking about becoming a coach, I got myself involved in the next stage, which was to stay embedded in this community. I thought about how I'd be a part of the community if I eventually became a coach, and I'd also be held more accountable. This had me keeping up the transformation and keep going with it.

After you've achieved your desired results, you should give yourself a treat. It could be anything at all. When I achieved my results, I booked myself a spa treatment as a personal reward for completing the WILDFIT Challenge. After the lovely spa, I had a nice and healthy lunch. It's part of just treating yourself and praising yourself for the hard work you've put in. You could for a meal or go to the movies. You could also go away on a short trip – maybe even a hike.

Try new things

You might realise you want to try new things after all these changes. I did that – I climbed the Sydney Harbour Bridge. This was something I'd always wanted to do, something adventurous. I'd never really had the courage to do it before, but I said, *"If I could achieve the result I have achieved with WILDFIT, what else can't I do?"*

So I booked myself in for a Harbour Bridge climb. It was one of the most memorable experiences I've ever had. You're right on top and looking at the whole of Sydney. When I climbed the Harbour Bridge, I didn't feel I was afraid of heights, but then I had never climbed anything that high before. It's a beautiful view. If you're in Sydney and haven't climbed the Harbour Bridge, I recommend it – and if you're not in Sydney, you should give it a try when you visit.

Trying new things comes with courage — though there's nothing wrong with getting a spa treatment or getting your hair done either. You want to give yourself the reward you deserve as part of your celebrations. It can just be something small. You might take a thirty-minute nap, have some me-time, or try meditation. It could also be a short walk while appreciating nature.

To continue my transformation journey, I've recently decided to take cooking classes. I'm learning how to make sushi and barbecues. For me, it's more about understanding the technique. As I said, I have not been trained as a professional cook or chef. I am trying to get a little more professional about it so I can properly enjoy my newfound lifestyle. This is really about living the lifestyle you've achieved while working on your new goal. You should know there's always the next level.

So what happens if you're not one hundred percent where you want to be?

You need to continue to refine the steps and work towards it, as you're very close. Keep track of your wins and gains. Celebrate the progress. Progress is the key to happiness. Sometimes, it's about the journey, not the destination.

I always feel there are certain areas I can improve in. Sometimes you might slip up, but if this happens you can always go back to step 2 and 3 of the framework. Then you just get back on track and keep going and moving in the right direction. The direction is more important.

If you go back to your journals and read over them from twelve months ago, you'll find that you've completely changed because of the transformation. It's about embracing who you are and who you've become. At this stage, it is really about you enjoying the fruit of your labour. You've done the hard work, and you've got the results you want. What you want to do is celebrate, accelerate and think about what's next.

Where do I want to go next time I achieve the desired results?

You should treat yourself, and treat yourself well. You don't want to go back to treating yourself like you used to in the past. Don't give yourself poor treats — giving yourself good treats after achieving results is a win, and builds your self-esteem.

When my clients had a graduation party after partaking in the transformation challenge, I advised them to list all their wins. Sometimes, the best wins were just getting back with a sense of control in your life. Another win is having extra energy, being able to go up and down the stairs without being puffed out. One of my clients was free of arthritis pain. She lost about thirty inches overall around her whole body. You can imagine how much mobility and flexibility that gave her. It's about having a clear mind to think about what you want next.

After getting your health right, making sure your nutrition is good and your food is healing and nourishing. Your body will be getting the correct fuel it needs to help you have a clear, focused mind. This will help you think about what you want to achieve next.

Enjoy this stage. This is all about Xtra acceleration, Xtra celebration and Xtra success. Give yourself the best chance to succeed and keep being part of the community of people that supported you, your role models. Think about how you can step up and share this message widely with the rest of the world. That's what this step is about. That wraps up the seventh and final step of the P.H.O.E.N.I.X. Framework.

Activity 9

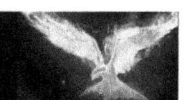

Make a list and schedule at least one small and one big reward/celebration (no limit here) to celebrate the progress you have made. Give yourself a reward for each goal that you have made progress with.

	List of rewards/celebration planned or scheduled
Goal 1.	
Goal 2.	
Goal 3.	

Chapter 10

Phoenix Rising – My Call to Be a WILDFIT Coach

"Sometimes you hear a voice through the door calling you. This turning towards what you deeply love saves you." - Rumi.

I was guided towards looking at this coaching opportunity. I had a full-time job. I just felt I needed to do more with the transformation I had undergone with WILDFIT in my health journey.

Being a coach comes with an association with the same community and having accountability. More importantly, stepping up and sharing this message around the world became my priority. My message was becoming clear. As soon as I saw that there was a master class about becoming a coach, I decided to attend it. I guess the best way to reinforce your learning is to share what you've learnt with others. Even if it seems impossible, you need to find a way. The reward at the other side is greater, and you lean more into mastery.

I felt that was what I needed to do to go further into my WILDFIT journey. People who stop participating and being part of the community will forget what they have learnt and go back to their old ways and behaviours. You don't want that to happen to you.

For me, becoming a coach was deeply personal. It came at a time when I only had a single income source, and being a single mother I wanted to establish multiple income streams.

I felt I had nothing permanent to fall back on if something were to happen to my job.

When this coaching opportunity came along, and I saw the results in my life, I decided that this was super important, and it was a guided message to be part of this community. I wondered how I could find a way to do it. It was a big commitment financially to pay for the coaching certification program, as I had existing commitments around my mortgage. I knew that funds were going to be really tight. I knew I'd have to cut expenses and other areas of my life. Well, I was delighted to make changes if it meant I could make that commitment to the coaching program. I was guided to go forward and do the WILDFIT coaching certification, so I found a way to find the finances for the program.

Before I finally decided to partake in the program, I went back and forth with my decision. Sometimes, when you're stuck between a rock and a hard place, you'll be confused about the next step to take. *If I do this, it will be hard – but if I do that, it's hard, too. What will I choose?* It's a tough decision. But I got logical about it, and used a decision making app to write down the pros and cons of my decisions. I needed to appeal to the rational, logical part of myself. You can do this as well. I went back to my purpose, and made sure I paid that investment fee for the coaching certification. I finally did it.

I had a great conversation with someone from WILDFIT and worked out a plan. I said, "Yes," and I think it's one of the best decisions that I've ever made. The moment I learnt about my health and transformation after becoming a coach, I'd reached yet another level. I could see the transformation and phoenix rising within me.

We are all spiritual beings, and we are all here with a purpose. Realising your purpose is up to you. After various experiences, like my brother's passing, my health issues and relationships, I felt I was here to serve a bigger purpose and help others.

Stepping up

Sometimes, people tell me I am inspiring, and things like that really made me step up. You just have to take the opportunity when it comes. There had been so many other opportunities I had looked at. I could have done some courses and other things, but the impact WILDFIT had on me is immeasurable.

After the program, I physically became different, and I could tell I had changed for the better. I could tell that this was my path, and it would be a privilege to help others the same way that WILDFIT had helped me. The pleasure I get every time I lead a group of people and see the results is immeasurable.

I remember week six or seven of my class, when I almost lost one of my clients. She told me that she wanted to give up on the challenge as she was going through some personal struggle with the breakup of a relationship. I asked her some questions and watched her make a decision to get back into it, because I'd made her remember her purpose in why she was doing WILDFIT in the first place. She went on to lose about ten kilos, and regained her confidence as she had never been that slim. She got back into clothes that she hadn't been able to fit into.

I knew that I had made the right decision – especially when I started seeing the results my clients were getting. It was just amazing to be of service to people. Everyone I've coached through WILDFIT so far has been so positive about the part I've played in their transformation. That is what life is about – it's about service, and being able to serve at the highest level, aligned with your highest purpose.

My mission became very clear. I decided I want to help one million people to improve their health. I know it's a massive number of people, but I can help them directly or indirectly. That's one of the reasons I decided to write this book. It's about getting the message out there so more people will know that there is help. You don't have to feel you're alone because there are so many people out there who have the answers. We've done the work and the research. That's my journey, and I'm still on it.

Meeting new challenges

It's been six months since I've completed the certification, and now it's a new challenge in figuring out how to get my message across. How do I grow my business organically? It's about how I help more people.

In one of my previous chapters, I said the trial class almost didn't happen, and that this journey almost didn't happen. I wouldn't have been able to help all the people I've helped. Well, I found a way, and I stuck to it. It was like my belief around it shifted. Of all the challenges I faced with finances, getting up early and showing up to the process, I just had to find a way to get several people together. It's really about getting clear with what you're focusing on.

- *Are you focusing on it working?* **Your focus should be on your belief that this is possible for you because you've put in the valuable investment.**

- *Will you see it through?* **For me, that's one of my values. When I decide to do something, I'll make sure I see it through. However, I may not get the exact results I want, but I never give up.**

Seeing it through

I am a chess player, and I started learning chess from a very young age. I competed at state tournaments, and I really did well. At a stage in a tournament, I played against a very good player, and she burst into tears during the match. She said she found me quite a formidable opponent, and she asked me to draw the game. Now, that was a game I was actually winning. I almost said "okay," because I felt sorry for her when she was crying. But I told myself it was a game and that we need to play the game to the end. That is what it is to be committed to something.

You need to do some research on what interests you, then schedule and lock things in. If you research and find something you want to pursue that will help you grow, then you could organise an appointment to meet with someone from that company to find out more about what that business offers.

For example, you might want to improve your mindfulness and you realise that you really want to try Tai-chi. You could research places that offer these classes in your area and see if you can book in for a trial class. You might give the Tai-chi place a call and find out more about their classes.

You won't lose, and you'll learn something in that half an hour. You might learn that you don't want to do it or learn that you're really curious about it. I urge you to step in and hear what your heart is saying. Your heart knows the way, and you need to run in that direction. You are not meant to crawl. You have wings, so learn to use them. When nothing is ventured, nothing is gained. You need to do this to really step into your power.

What if you can't do it anymore?

There will always be things that are not in your sphere of influence. Say you are injured, or you found something that isn't in your control. In this case, try not to worry about what you can't control. You can only control your own behaviour and actions, not the actions of others. You can influence them to an extent if they're open to it – but you cannot control it fully, so don't waste time trying to do that. Change how you respond to it and remain true to yourself.

It's about aligning to your true purpose with your mind, body and soul. What's the point of living with superficial and materialistic things when there's so much more you can discover at a deeper level?

Activity 10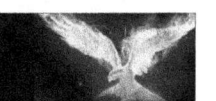

As an exercise for you, think about something in your life that's calling you to step up. It could be one of those areas you feel is not where it should be or that's bugging you. Choose an area that's important to you, but maybe you have not been able to get traction in it. See how you can commit

Area	Things/Projects/classes I am inspired to do

What if you don't know your wish or your mission?

The main reason you're reading this book is that you feel you have a bigger purpose. Otherwise, you wouldn't have picked up this book. You are doing really well, so well done.

Your mission will come to you at the right time. Just do the work, and the answer will come from within you. Where is your biggest pain point or concerns? Which struggles in your life come with a little annoyance? That is where the answers lie. After answering these questions, you'll know what your mission is. Don't stress about it. Just continue to do the work, show up, and you'll see it happen.

Chapter

11

Boost The Lives of Others, One Person at a Time

"Be a lamp, or a lifeboat, or a ladder. Help someone's soul heal."- Rumi.

One of the biggest reasons I decided to be a coach was that it feels really good when I help others. You will feel the same if you help others achieve their goals. You become a part of the 'high vibe tribe' and live your full potential when you do things that are in service to others.

I once went to a Zumba class where the instructor was starting a new class. It was a new business and a new place. Two people showed up for the first class, but I won't forget what happened after that. The instructor gave their best, like they would if fifty people were present. The energy was intense.

That taught me that even if one person shows up to your class, you should give them your 100%. You should still show up, and do everything you can to help that person. Sometimes that might be difficult to do. Your morale might be affected when you don't have the turn-up you expected, but you have got to show up for the people who have come to the class. When people don't show up, it's not like they don't like you. Don't take things personally. They just have other stuff to do. Don't take things personally if someone doesn't say thank you for your help, get back to you, or even give you much credit. It's fine as long as you've delivered your side of the bargain. Your part is to give value, and you've done that.

You should show up with the same awesome energy and commitment you would put in if one hundred people were present. Even if you make a difference to just one person's life, you're doing a lot more than if you weren't making any difference at all. How do you know that one person won't go out and help another thousand people? The value of helping one person shouldn't be underestimated.

We're all go-getters, but I think we should all be *go-givers* because there's an amazing feeling that comes with giving. The joy that comes with seeing people happy after you've helped them through a tough decision or phase is what life is about. That is what serving is about, and I believe that's what I'm doing here.

I feel if you're not following you life's purpose, you simply exist in life and you are not fully alive. When you live on purpose, there's a sense of mission or vision when you get out of bed in the morning. You always feel that work needs to be done, and there's excitement and pleasure that comes from within because you think there is something bigger than you. When you don't live on purpose, every day just feels like another day – another day without a mission. You'd just say, *"Let me just stay in. I don't have anything that matters enough."* That's the message you're sending to your brain, and that's not very nice because you are here to deliver a higher purpose.

Hopefully, this book has given you some ideas and inspiration to find your purpose, and realise what your goals and commitments could be or look like in the next three to twelve months. If you don't do the inner work to find out those answers, you won't be living on purpose.

Pointing in the right direction

One of the reasons I wrote this book is to get the message out that there are answers to your questions. Some people have done the research and work, got answers, and they can help you.

The first group I coached in WILDFIT was a small one, but I still showed up and helped. Whenever I deal and interact with one person, they should feel like they're in a better position as a result of that interaction. God knows what their day was like before you came onto the scene.

You can be that person who makes a difference in someone's life. It doesn't only have to be while you're coaching or doing your work. Every time you talk or connect with someone, you have an opportunity to help them, and that's exactly what I do. I try to give the kind of energy I want to see in someone else. I also try to give that to people who are not feeling strong. I was like that some time ago, and I might be that person again at a different point in my life. My point is that, wherever you can, you should try to boost the lives of others. Show up in every interaction you have.

When I'm having these conversations about WILDFIT with people, I am not looking at what I can sell them. It's never that way for me. It's like we are talking right now – we're having an interaction. I always want to understand before I tell you what the solution is. I want to understand your goals and why they're important to you, because I want to work with people I can help. If I can't help you, then I would say, *"Sorry, I don't think I can help you. I think you're better off trying something else."*

You don't want to be pushing yourself onto someone if you are not the right person to help them. Give them other resources or recommend other people who might be able to help. For instance, someone spoke to me the other day, and I went through their health goals and tried to understand what was important to them.

She told me, "Oh, I want to be fifty kilos. I just want to be fifty kilos."

She wanted to know if I had some protein shakes and milkshakes to give her. I felt that was not something I could help her with. At WILDFIT, we have different ways of doing things. We go back to the basics. It's about going back to nature and see what's available. So I told her she was better off trying something else. She didn't sign up, and that was fine.

I try to avoid making promises I can't deliver on or saying I can help when I can't. I can probably get you where you want to be, but I need you to put in the time, commitment and be open to the way the challenge works. Always be upfront and honest about your intention and where you're coming from.

Self-care and showing up

I think for you to serve others, you also need to show up for yourself. I believe self-care is really important, and that's something I learnt when I became a mother. Being a first-time mum, I asked myself who would take care of my child if I was sick. I was thinking about everybody else's needs first, and that wasn't going to work. If you really want to serve at a high level and step into your purpose, you need to look after yourself. You can't care for others if you don't care for yourself.

People will see the standards you set for yourself. You want to be authentic and be in a place where you can truly give without resentment and regrets. You need to care for yourself and boost your life to do that. You need to keep learning, improving, growing and contributing to your core values as there's always something new to learn, some area you can improve in.

Once you get to this stage, make a list of who you can help. Be clear on what you want to do and what your mission is. You might be surprised when those on your list approach you. We're all energy; everything is frequency and energy – so, if you think about them, they start moving closer to you.

If you're reading this book and feel this will help you, I would love to connect with you. If you know other people who can also benefit from this framework, you can help them by recommending this book. When I can't help someone, I give them a contact of the person in the best position to help. That's a part of directly or indirectly boosting other people's lives.

Think about your message. What is it you stand for?

When you get clear on your message, you attract the right people who you can help. Getting clear on my message is something I spend a lot of time thinking about. Once I got that sorted, I was really clear on who I wanted to help, and those people were the ones who were attracted to the book or attracted to the coaching programs I was doing.

After reading this book, think about how you can share your key message. Make a list of people you can help and serve. Once you get to that stage where you feel your phoenix has risen and you want to deliver more value to other people's lives, you should take it from there. I believe that's what we're here to do.

No one can do what you can do because you are unique, and there is only one of you. Even though there are thousands of books written about transformation, nobody has written this book because it is mine. Now, I feel I have some key messages to share. Think about your own key messages, and what you've been yearning for all your life. I wish you good luck with that journey.

Boost The Lives of Others, One Person at a Time

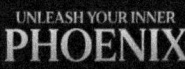 # Activity 11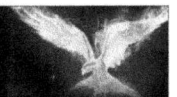

List your key messages that you are inspired and curious about, and pay attention to this.

	What are you getting curious or inspired to do?
1.	
2.	
3.	
4.	
5.	

Chapter 12

Spark Action for Your Success

"It's your road and yours alone. Others may walk it with you, but no one can walk it for you."- Rumi.

Apply the framework. Be a practitioner in your own life. That is my earnest wish for you. Otherwise, this would be just another book you bought to put on your shelf. Hopefully I've given you enough examples of how an ordinary person like me can change and transform their life after going through experiences that have been quite painful. I don't know you personally, but what I do know is that if you've taken the time to read this book, the next step is to take massive action on whatever it is you need to do.

This is the moment to apply the P.H.O.E.N.I.X. Framework. I'd love to hear the stories of how you applied it. If you want to connect with me on my Instagram or Facebook page, I would love to hear from you and hear your stories.

What are the benefits of taking action?

Obviously you will get results. You have learnt a framework, and the application of this framework will change your life for the better, and you'll have more fulfilment.

Live life like everything is rigged in your favour. Run from what's comfortable, because being comfortable means nothing has changed. If it's an uncomfortable feeling, that means you're changing and there is some growth happening. Otherwise, you'll be stuck in your comfort zone and stuck with your pain.

You have your dreams. You're facing your fears and taking action. Don't let fear stop you. Fear is an emotion, and it needs to be processed. It is your fear, and you need to take responsibility for it. You have to face it, then have the courage to move forward. You don't have to take a massive huge action at first. You can just take a little step. You need to take small consistent actions and you need to show up every day and keep going. For example, say there's a big meal you want to eat, and it is a good quality organic meal. You won't eat the whole meal in one go. You'll break it down into small pieces or steps first.

You should also never leave an event or situation without making a decision to go further. For example, you may have just heard an amazing talk about the benefits of exercise, and you realise it would be great for you to start exercising. Right there and then in that moment, complete one small action that will ensure you follow through with the next step. It could be scheduling time in your calendar to do a workout, or making a call to go and check out the nearby gym.

It all starts with the right mental state, mindset and good daily rituals. Make sure your daily rituals are in your calendar, like drinking a lot of water, deep breathing and meditation. I also do some exercises to get me in the right mood and set my goals for the day. I ensure my daily success by keeping myself in a peak state mentally, emotionally and physically.

Join me on this journey

Having read this book, I'm sure you'll realise your actions need to be taken in small steps. There is a big difference between cognitively understanding something and trying to understand it in practice. You may have got tips and ideas from what I've been telling you, but it's time to fully engage as I did for the 90-Day WILDFIT Challenge.

As a WILDFIT coach, I am offering to coach anyone who has read this book and take them through the WILDFIT 90-Day Challenge, which is a food psychology and nutrition-based program. I coach clients to help them with their health and food relationships. I can also offer you an opportunity to try WILDFIT for two weeks, where you'll get practical experience. That's what you need for true transformation to happen at a cellular level. There is no wrong action – there's just action that you learn from and get results from. You just course-correct and keep going.

There is a candle in your heart that is ready to be kindled if you've read this far. There is a voice in your soul, and it's ready to be heard. You hear the voice, don't you? I have given you a framework you can apply. Use the templates I recommend and the tips and insights I've shared with you from my experience. If you apply that, you will get the desired results. I did, and it worked for me.

You need to go back and reflect on what you've learnt from this book. I would love for you to write down your top three takeaways as soon as you finish reading the book while it's still fresh in your mind.

Come visit my website (details at the start of the book), and find out how I can help you if your health is one of your goals. I would love to serve you. Get in touch with me to schedule a health unpack appointment, where we'll go through your health goals and work out if WILDFIT is the right fit for you. Then take action. You need to take every little step.

Make the change

When people say they want to make some changes in their lives, time and money are two basic things that might hinder them from pursuing that change. If you channel the time and energy you spend on dealing with your pain into applying this framework, you will free up a lot of energy. I manage my energy, and when your energy is managed, you can get better results from anything you do.

For instance, I could have made the excuse that I didn't have enough money to do the WILDFIT certification, but I didn't because I knew the program was important to me. I found the resources. It's not always about the resources – it's about how resourceful you are to reach your goals. If you can't do it straight away, make a plan – or at least take a small step towards it. That itself will send a direct message, saying, *"Okay, there is some level of commitment here."* Then you need to take another step consistently in that direction.

Get really clear on what you're doing. Use activities I've mentioned in this book. Do your meditations and look at your daily processes. Check if your daily actions are actually helping you move towards the life you visualise. If they are not helping, do a *Start, Stop, Continue* exercise. *Start* what you need to do. *Stop* doing what is not serving you, and *Continue* what is working for you. Once you manage your energy and make the Start, Stop, Continue list, then you can review your goals.

You have done all this inner work and got all your answers from within. Then you can make a plan towards fulfilling your goal. Taking action is the best way to learn. Sometimes, you have to fire the shot when you're not fully ready, because taking that shot makes you see what went well and what you could do differently. Just try to work it out and figure it out in your head.

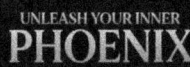 # Activity 12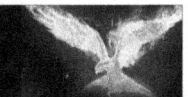

Pick a goal that you want to review using the Start, Stop, Continue exercise.

Things I could start doing	Things I should stop doing	Things I should continue doing

Activity 13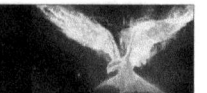

List three to five actions you can take now to schedule and progress towards your goals.

	Action List
1.	
2.	
3.	
4.	
5.	

I strongly urge you to use this book to spark massive action, and I want you to take consistent steps towards your goal. It doesn't stop. Yes, it's a journey. Yes, you're headed towards a destination. Yes, you must celebrate your progress so far. You must celebrate all your successes, but you do need to take action.

My biggest belief I had to shift was saying, *"No, I'm not ready."* I used to procrastinate a lot, and it made me miss out on opportunities. I did not procrastinate about doing the 90-Day WILDFIT Challenge. I did deliberate over it, but I did not procrastinate from doing it.

I'd love you to take action and implement all the things you have worked out through the activities in the book. I can help you with the implementation if health is your goal and if you have any questions.

I am happy to share my stories. I am constantly sharing messages via my website and social media pages on Instagram, Facebook and LinkedIn. I would love to hear from you. If there's something I can do to help, then please reach out.

I wish you all the very best with your journey. Thank you for taking the time to join me in in *Unleashing Your Inner Phoenix*.

I would love to see your unleashed version. I would love to hear from you.

Take care and keep me posted. Thank you.

Love and best wishes,
Kaveri

Acknowledgements

There are many people who have helped me along the way in my journey. This book is dedicated to everyone in my professional and personal life who have played a part in bringing me to this point in my journey. It is also dedicated to my parents, who have done the best they can for me and given me unconditional love always.

I am very grateful to Eric Edmeades and WILDFIT for helping me with my transformation.

In my professional life I would to thank Miriam Silva, who is the epitome of what a leader looks like! Her support, guidance and support during my initial years in Australia is something I will never forget. Miriam is one of a kind, and I am just so lucky that our paths crossed.

I would also like to thank Sue Woodhead, who has been a terrific mentor to me in my Change Management career, and has been a pillar of strength every day since.

Thank you to Christine Artin, Tara Yates and Vicki Mitrevska for the role they played in helping me secure some of my first change management roles! Thankyou Genevieve Looney and Ann-Maree Lawrence, who have been amazing people to work for. I really feel very valued and respected in the team.

There are too many others to name, and rest assured I am very grateful for all of you and the roles you have played.

In my personal life, I would like to thank Shanthie De Mel for helping me in my very first weeks in Australia with warm food and a blanket! I was not prepared for Melbourne winter! I would also like to thank Annette Briggs for being an amazing supporter and friend, especially in our first few years in Australia! She is a rock and a pillar of strength, and I am so lucky to know you.

I would like to thank Avril Hurtis for being like a sister, my closest friend and confidant over my years in Australia. We are practically like family! So lucky to have your generosity of spirit in my life.

Thank you Krithika Kumar Quintal, my dearest friend from school, who has been there for me through thick and thin. She even flew to Australia in 2018 for my 40th birthday and made it so special. She is someone who is a constant in my life.

Thank you to Nive Chelaka (and her sister Nisha, too), who is another dear friend of mine from school and university. She followed me to Australia, and is also there for me when I need emotional support.

I would like to thank Sara Kulk, my Zumba bestie. You helped me so much when I was going through a touch patch in my life after my separation – not just with Zumba, but also with my health. She was in fact my first health coach, and I learnt a lot from her.

My beautiful friends Lizzy Van Dalen and Samara Borges, who I met on my birthday in 2020. We knew then that we were going to be friends for a long time.

There are so many more friends from school, university, and work mates who became friends – too many to name here. I thank you one and all.

My brother Ashwin, who passed away at 22. I thank you for being an awesome brother and showing me what it is like to have a sibling. He was calm and wise for his young age. I miss you every day.

And my extended family, who I have reconnected with after a long time. It's been so cathartic and wonderful. Thank you all so much.

I love you all.

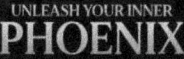
UNLEASH YOUR INNER PHOENIX

Table of Value	SILVER	GOLD	PLATINUM
Unpack Health Goals for client			
Health Game changer Calls with a certified WILDFIT Coach to get clarity on health goals and check for right fit	✓	✓	✓
3 take-aways to get stated on your journey	✓	✓	✓
TRY WILDFIT			
Video coaching Program - daily for 2 weeks	✓	✓	✓
6 coaching calls with Certified WILDFIT coach in a group	✓	✓	✓
Awareness on Mindset and Psychology around food	✓	✓	✓
Nutrition guidance to help body to reset	✓	✓	✓
Awareness on different types of hungers	✓	✓	✓
Access to Private Facebook community	✓	✓	✓
Recording of all coaching calls made available within 24 hours	✓	✓	✓
WILDFIT 90-Day Challenge			
12 weeks video coaching program (TRY WILDFIT is the first 2 weeks)		✓	✓
Bi-weekly group coaching calls with Certified WILDFIT coach		✓	✓
Access to Private Facebook community		✓	✓
Mindset coaching for food psychology & to better understand food relationships		✓	✓
3 check-ins for measurements to track progress		✓	✓
Access to coach via private Facebook community through the week		✓	✓
Coaching through the weekly enhancements during the challenge		✓	✓
Safe environment to move through any tough parts of the challenge		✓	✓
Recording of all coaching calls made available within 24 hours		✓	✓
Celebrating wins at a graduation party		✓	✓
BONUS			
Free Q&A session about the P.H.O.E.N.I.X. Framework			✓
Free WILDFIT coaching support calls x3 after the challenge			✓
Free Meditations for inner calm			✓

Notes

Unleash your inner Phoenix

Notes

Unleash your inner Phoenix

Notes

Unleash your inner Phoenix

Notes

Unleash your inner Phoenix

Notes

Unleash your inner Phoenix

Notes

Unleash your inner Phoenix

Notes

Unleash your inner Phoenix

Notes

Unleash your inner Phoenix

Notes

Unleash your inner Phoenix

Notes

Unleash your inner Phoenix

Notes

www.ingramcontent.com/pod-product-compliance
Lightning Source LLC
Chambersburg PA
CBHW081352080526
44588CB00016B/2464